HEALTH EQUALS WEALTH

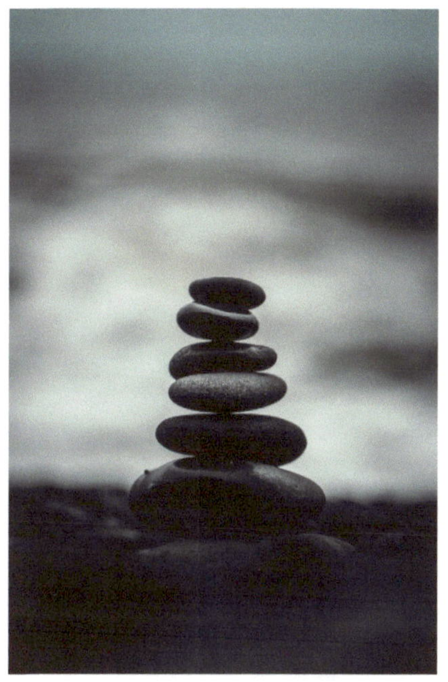

by Natalija Russell

CONTENTS

Copyright © 2023 Natalija Russell

All rights reserved

The characters and events portrayed in this book are fictitious. Any similarity to real persons, living or dead, is coincidental and not intended by the author.

No part of this book may be reproduced, or stored in a retrieval system, or transmitted in any form or by any means, electronic, mechanical, photocopying, recording, or otherwise, without express written permission of the publisher.

For More Information:

wisefeather369@gmail.com
or go to
www.wise-feather.com

ISBN:
Imprint: Independently Published

Cover design by: Robert Russell

"Health is not valued till sickness comes"

THOMAS FULLER

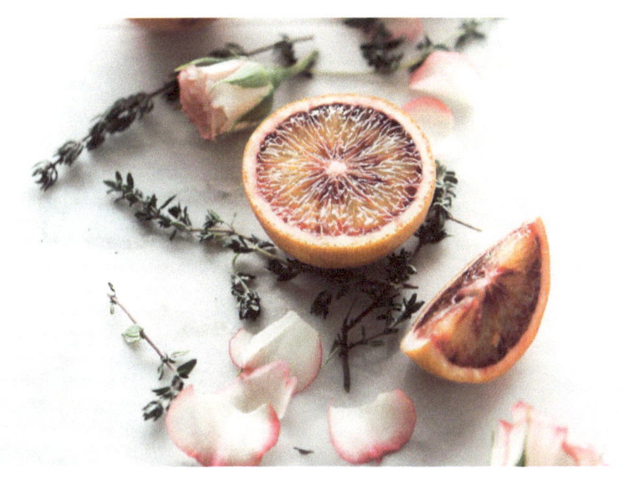

INTRODUCTION

I am writing this booklet in hope that it will serve and help other people on their health journey. It was not just physical but also a very spiritual journey that took a lot from me.

Sometimes we don't know what we have until its gone. But on that journey, I have learned so much about myself.

How to love myself, how to take care of me first and how to set priorities and boundaries in my life.

Now I know that I come first and everything else can wait.

I have also learned how to listen to my own body and its needs and how to set routines that are beneficial for me and my wellbeing.

I trust that this little booklet gives you hope and inspires you on your own health journey or that its serves as a

cautionary tale.
We don't always have to learn from our own mistakes, we can learn from other people to.

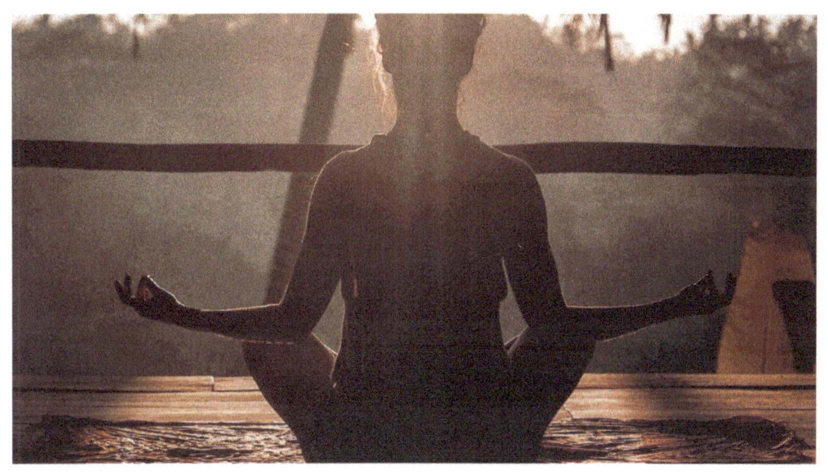

HEALTH IS WEALTH, WISE PEOPLE WOULD SAY....

We so often take it for granted and then, when something happens to us, and we lose it we tend to think that that's just how it works.

Everything is energy and so is your health. If it's flowing, you are at ease and if not, you are creating dis-ease.

Disease is blocked energy trapped inside of your body that needs to get out. The longer its inside more damage it will create. And eventually it will manifest itself outside or inside of your body as an illness of some kind.

It's all done to our blocked emotions. When things happen in our life, instead of going with the flow excepting things as they are, we tend to fight it, get angry, frustrated, sad and then those emotions we don't let through our bodies.

We tend to bury them, pretend that they are not there by eating more, drinking, or doing anything just so that we would not feel and face them.

Because no one like to feel bad do they?

And after a while those same emotions start to create problems in our lives, creating various diseases and we are totally oblivious to what is happening and that we ourselves are responsible for what we have created unconsciously. We have so much power but have never been taught how to use it to benefit from it in our life's.

It starts with the mental plane because everything is mental in this universe.

Your thoughts have power and if you don't learn how to use that power, you will get abused by it.

And that is exactly what we humans tend to do.

Every thought you have is creative, it is a binding tissue of this reality, and we create our own reality with our thoughts along with co-creating on the collective level as well. Power of our mind is so great, and we need to learn how to guide it to where we want to go, and not allow to be guided by it.

We need to learn to use our minds and think for ourselves, because if we don't, we just become a part of a heard, collective thinking and we just repeat what everyone else is thinking, which manifests in doing what everyone else is doing. Illness starts in the mind first and it creates the environment where it festers.

Beware of your thoughts and learn how to think properly.

By focusing on what you don't want to happen, you call it in, because where your thoughts go energy flows.
The more you feed into negative thinking, the more of it you will receive cause the universe does not give you what you want.

Universe responds to your feelings and that is the secret. The more you learn how to master your emotions the better your life and health will be.
Work on yourself is the greatest gift you can give yourself and others and your life will never be the same.
Someone said you will either pay the farmer or the doctor and I know that is the greatest truth about your health. You will either look after it and be grateful you have it, or you will lose it and pay to try and get it back.

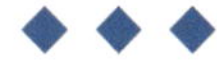

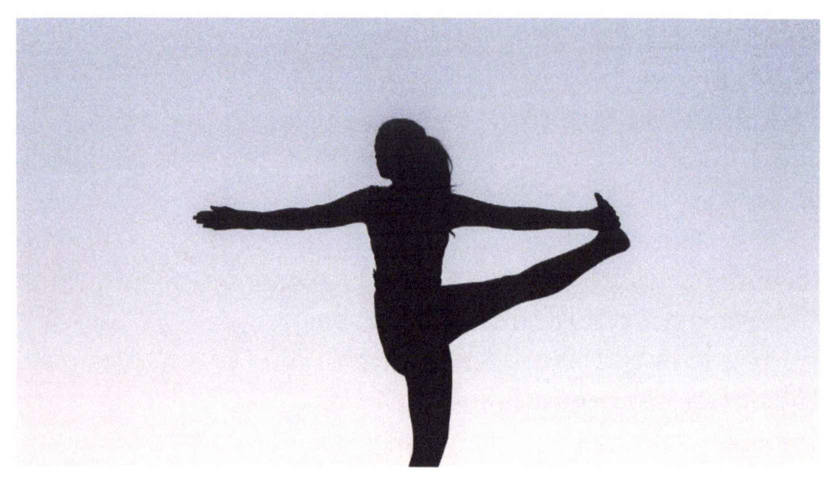

APPRECIATE YOUR HEALTH WHILE YOU HAVE IT

Your health is the most underestimated thing in the world. At least I thought that about my own health. I was young in my thirties, so called best years of my life.

I had no issues, pains, or any sort of problems with my health.

I didn't even think about my health because I had other things on my mind.

I had my hopes and dreams to fulfil, my family to look after and my son to raise.

So many other things were on my mind that health wasn't even on the back of it.

After a while life started to be a bit more intense but I thought that's just how it is, we all have issues and difficulties, and nobody is exempt from it so just deal with it.

I was a problem solver and always so busy with achieving my goals and plans that, I never had the time to stop and listen to my body, take a break, and do some self-care.

I would do everything for everyone without even a question asked, people pleaser for sure.

I was always giving to others but not to myself first, but after a while my cup was empty and there was nothing to give any more. I also realised that no one was giving to me. Where are all this people now, when I need them?

Why is no one asking how I am?

It didn't take me long to figure out I was out of balance. Not in that moment when it was all happening but now with this awareness, I know I was.

The biggest proof that I was out of balance was when life put me down by breaking my foot in two places so I couldn't move for next 3 months.

That was a sign from above to slow down and then I realised even when I am not forcing things to happen and putting a lot of effort, things would still manifest, just in a different way. I would just attract them to me anyway.

Life was trying to tell me that in different ways, but I didn't listen.

I didn't know that then, but I was mostly in my masculine

energy.   We all have both jinn/feminine and Jang/ masculine energies within us. If they are not balanced out within us, we will be out of balance.

That is how you get people who are constantly action driven, overworked, and burned out, or on the other side of the coin the ones who never finish anything because they are always procrastinating.

We need both energies to be balanced and to learn how to go with the flow of life and not listen to what society has been teaching us, and that is to constantly go and do things.

There is a time for inspired action but also a time to wait until things come to you by you being in your feminine energy and attracting things to yourself.

I must say as a woman I was taught from early on to be more in masculine -action driven energy. I have learned to suppress my emotions because there were a weakness in a society I grew up.

Of course, It took me years to relearn everything I have been programmed with, a lot of self-help books, tremendous amount of work on myself and my character.

Diving deep into my shadow self and working on changing my belief system and transforming into a person I am today. It wasn't easy and I had no help from anyone just a big desire to change. Nothing was making sense in my life, and I was questioning my reality daily.

I would go out and just observe people around me, strangers and the one I already knew.

I always had this knowing within me that there was more to life than what meets the eye and that I don't want to have stupid shallow conversations with people.

I also didn't want to waste mine or other peoples time because time is all we have.

Now I know that that knowing was my intuition all along.

I was very stubborn and would not listen there fore would have to learn some of the life lessons the hard way. And that was exactly what happen to me.

I did not get a terminal illness, but an auto-immune disease called psoriasis.

Basically, your skin cells die of to quickly forming plaque on your skin which can be itchy and painful and let's not forget very unsightly on the outside of your skin.

And let's be real here, it was not just the shear look of it that was so uncomfortable for me, it was suffering for sure.

My whole head and bits of my body were covered with patches that were bleeding and itching at the same time.

Then I realized my body was crying for help and that help was only the beginning of what was yet to come.

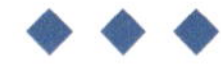

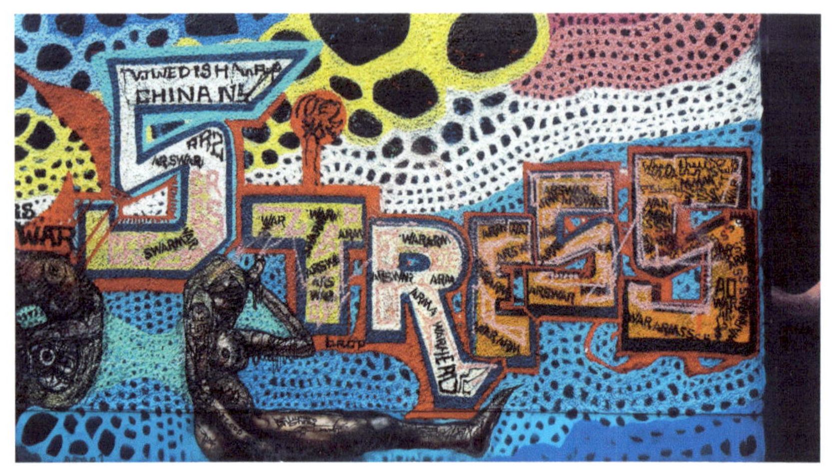

STRESS IS A KILLER

My illness was now deeply rooted in my reality showing me that my pain was so deep that it finally manifested in my physical reality.

I was shocked to realized how much I have put my body through. I was always the strong one, not paying any attention on the signs my body was showing me long before the manifestation of my illness.

Stress was real and it was killing me from the inside out.

Auto-immune means that your body is attacking itself.

Like I had a death wish deep within.

I have put myself in so much pain and suffering by not looking after myself properly and not seeing the signs on the way. It was devastating to see my skin in the state it was in, and I started to think and reflect deeply about my situation. I knew I have put myself in this predicament and I will get myself out of it. My outlook on life was always positive and optimistic and I knew I was going to keep the faith, and believe that things can and will improve, and that I can and will change my life and my health for the better.

My intuition was telling me that this was not just a case of treating the consequences but also dealing with the root cause of the problem.

For sure I am a very deep thinker, and this will go very deep into my subconscious mind to find why this was happening to me.

And what is it teaching me?

From my spiritual perspective the skin problem I had was on some level not feeling good in my own skin, in my own body, being me.

That was my root cause and I had to deal with it in my own way. Most people would see and talk to a psychologist and pay for years of therapy but not stubborn old me.

I have always been very independent, doing everything by myself from an early age.

I also love psychology and have studied it on my own accord for years.

I love to analyse people, look at their body language and pay attention on what they do and not what they say.

Most people are not authentic or in their integrity, so their words have no meaning or power.

What they do is everything because actions speak louder than words, how the saying goes.

My love of psychology led me to learn more about it and to dive deep within my subconscious mind where all our belief system is. Also working with my own shadow was probably the hardest but satisfying work that a person can give to themselves.

Integration has led me to many aha moments that made me see what I was doing and why.
I abused my body so much, not listening to all the signs it was giving me. I apologise for that.
I am not my body; I have a body.
And my body made me ill to finally start paying attention to it. It was a cry for help for sure.
I realised my body is my temple, vehicle of my soul and it's on me to love it, look after it and take care of it and it will serve me for many years to come.
Then I decided to change.

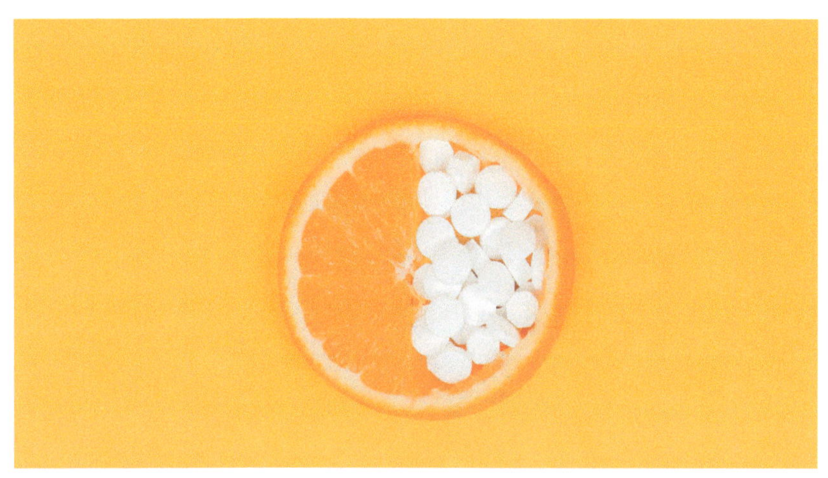

LONG PATH OF RECOVERY

For four years I was exposing myself to stress, that was having a terrible effect on my mental and physical health.

In the process of me striving for my dreams and goals I lost sight of what really mattered, and that was my health. I kept telling myself I need to sacrifice for things that I wanted to achieve but I was totally unaware of the damage I was doing to myself.

Like a stubborn bull I can sometimes be (referring to my

astrological sign taurus), I just held my goals in front of me and wouldn't budge.

Now I know better and would not risk my health like that ever again. You live and you learn, I guess.

The road of recovery did start with a decision to change, on a physical, mental, and spiritual level.

I had to become a different personality to be able to create a new reality. Because the old me couldn't create anything new, I had to really go deep in my subconscious to the source of my belief system.

I had to know why I have created a skin problem.

Why didn't I feel good in my own skin?

Why was I hiding my true self?

Why wasn't I loving to myself?

Did I not feel worthy?

Wasn't I good enough?

Who made me think this way and where were these beliefs coming from. It was slow and painful facing certain things about myself that I have buried deep within but from this perspective, I have today I must say it was totally worth it. I had to change my own beliefs about myself and the best way to do that is to listen to affirmations about self-worth, self-love, and self-acceptance.

You can find them all over internet, books or even make your own. They are just positive statements that you repeat to yourself every day repeatedly. It is a process, and it will take some time and patience to see any results. You are planting new seeds in your mind, and it take time, love, effort for them to grow and show up in your life. So don't give up, all the good things in life are worth waiting for. I also had to pay extra attention on my inner voice.

My generation was mostly criticized growing up by our parents and authority and that voice becomes our inner critic, always telling us we are not good enough, pretty enough, not deserving and so on.

And this is not an invite to start hating and resenting your parents or your carers, but to truly understand that they did the best they could.

If they knew better, they would do better, in most cases.

So, you evolve and become a better person for yourself and your children. Every time we break the chains of our family line, we are freeing ourselves and the generations that were here before us.

It is evolution at its best.

There was a lot of clearing old beliefs, planting new ones, a lot of healing that had to occur and forgiveness that had to happen. Forgiving myself, my parents, people around me who hurt me and a lot of emotional clearing in general.

That's why a very good psychologist can be important link on your journey to recovery.

We all carry traumas from childhood and are not even aware of them and the effect they tend to hold on our life's. We create from our subconscious and that's why it is so important to know what is hidden there and bring it back to light.

Remember, we become illuminated by facing the dark first and then being the light.

That was my work on the mental and emotional plane.

I also had to work on my physical plane and the best way to start was from food. Food is medicine if you know what to eat to heal your body.

By process of elimination, I had to learn about my body and its preferences. I had to educate myself about what food is inflammatory and witch one wasn't. I had to figure out what was the best food for me and was it sustainable. I did not want to go on a diet as such, it was more of a lifestyle choice. I was learning how to feed my body with proper nutrients and to try and keep away from processed food that is not good.

The more colourful your plate the better for your health it is. Implementing vitamins that are beneficial for my health was crucial too.

Learning how to take care of my body, such as washing it with natural product and paying attention about different substances in care products such as shampoo, body wash, lotions, and shower gels.

It was a journey for sure.

Also learning how to set boundaries was a big one.

I tend to do so much for others because of my carrying nature but a lesson was learned that my cup must be filled first, and overflowing, only then I can give to others.

Balance between give and take was a big lesson too.

I was closed for receiving from others so I would naturally attract the takers in my life.

Now I know better. Another big thing on my journey was to stop and smell the roses. I stopped chasing and started to enjoy living in present moment. And being grateful for all I have in my life right now. That stopped my anxiety.

We only get anxious while worrying about the future and depressed by dwelling in the past so being present is paramount.

Meditation has helped me tremendously. It has helped me to calm the overactive mind I had and to find that peace within I was looking for.

Only when you create that peace within yourself, you can see it outside of you.

Because your outer world is only a projection of your inner world.

I stopped smoking after 23 years in that period which

helped with psoriasis.

I have included daily exercise and walking in my routine as a part of my new lifestyle.

I did not just want to use a cream prescribed from my doctor because I knew that it would only make me addicted for the rest of my life.

I wanted to be a new person and for that, I really had to change my personality so that my personal reality would change as well.

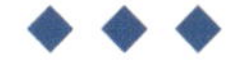

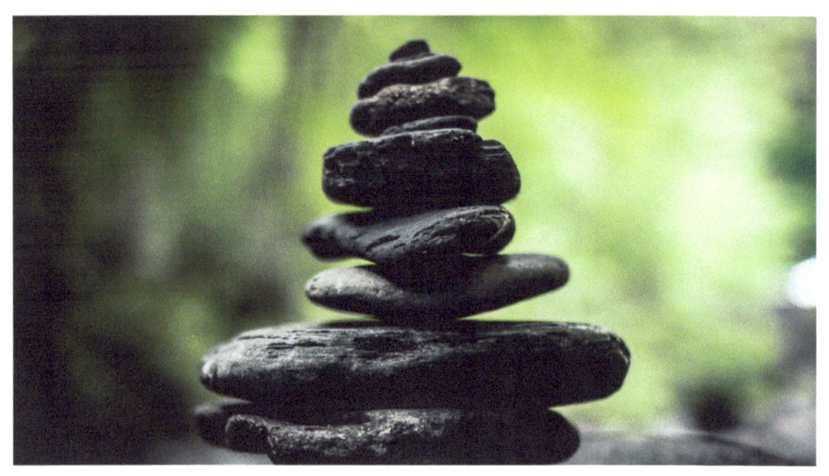

FINDING BALANCE WITHIN

For me finding balance within was mostly learning how to trust and let go.

Learning to go with the flow of life, having that faith and trust that things will work out for my highest good and the good of others.

Even without me having to control everything.

I must say that I was a bit of a control freak, and even though it is still within me, I have learned to keep a close eye on that freak, so it doesn't take over the reins of my life

ever again. Finding that balance within means that I am mostly learning to be in the receptive mode, in that jinn energy, which I sometimes find very hard to do.
But I m still learning and will be for years to come for sure.
Now I am very much aware of every aspect of my life weather that is health, work, friendships, or family.
I am very grateful for my experiences, even though they were hard on me.
I have learned so much and have gained so much wisdom from it that I have this to share with the world.
We all want the world to change but by changing ourselves the world changes as well.

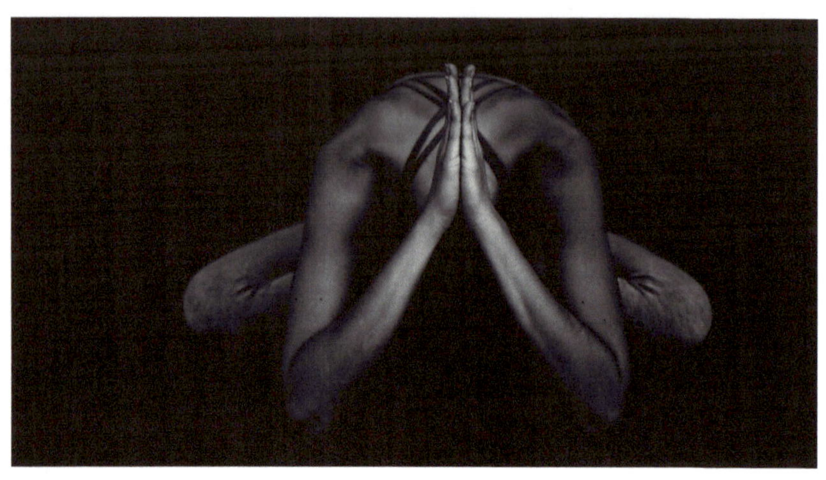

PRIORITISING YOUR HEALTH

For me that means that I treat my body with the up most respect.

It is my suit of armour, vehicle of my soul.

It is my temple and must be treated like that as well.

I still have a lot to do in that respect, for sure I am not a perfect being.

I make mistakes and hopefully learn from them.

But I am for sure more aware of my body, I know how to listen to it, how to feed it properly, how to treat it with love and care and be grateful for all that it does for me.

I am so blessed to have my health back.

And yes, psoriasis is gone, and my skin has been clear for a while but the lessons I have learned in this process are priceless.

You only realise what you got when its gone.

So, if you can, take the easy road and be grateful for it now.

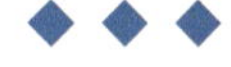

BOOKS BY THIS AUTHOR

Rainbow Warriors & The New Earth: A Guide To Conscious Living

From my own personal spiritual journey, I decided to write this guide to help any soul who wants to grow in state of consciousness and create their own heaven on earth.

Why Are Some People Poor? : And How To Become Wealthy

This little booklet is a blend of my own personal experiences and observations when it comes to money mentality. Hopefully it will serve you well as a guide to change your own.

Realisation Of Divine Within Me

This book describes my own personal growth and how I have changed from a low state of consciousness to a higher state. It also serves the reader as a guide on their own personal path.

What Are Friendships?: A Spiritual Perspective

I wrote this little booklet to describe to the reader what the true meaning of friendship really is.

From our human perspective they are just people we love to spend our time with, but from our soul perspective there is so much more that we can discover. This booklet is based on my own personal journey and its purpose is to give the reader insight and a new perspective on friendship.

From 3D To 5D: From Fear To Love - From Matter To Energy

This booklet is all about shifting into a new paradigm. Globally we are all shifting into a new state of consciousness and we are now in a place of transition from 3D to 5D, literally going from matter to energy. This comes from my own inner knowing and I invite you all on a journey of self discovery.

ABOUT THE AUTHOR

Natalija Russell

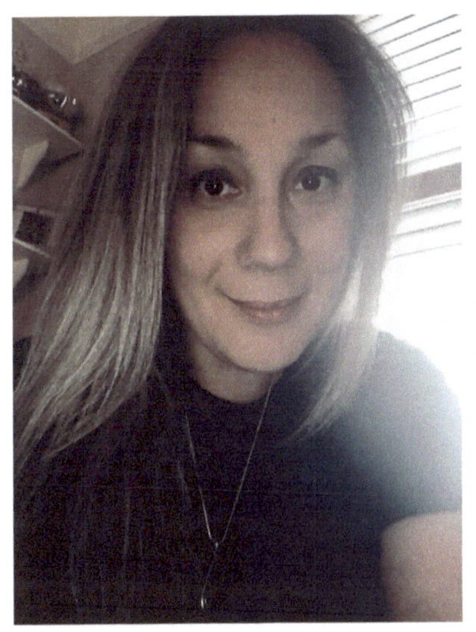

First and foremost, I am a mother and a wife, a spiritual coach and master life coach, singer and writer. A Woman who took her own spiritual journey and transformed her life...... "May you do the same"